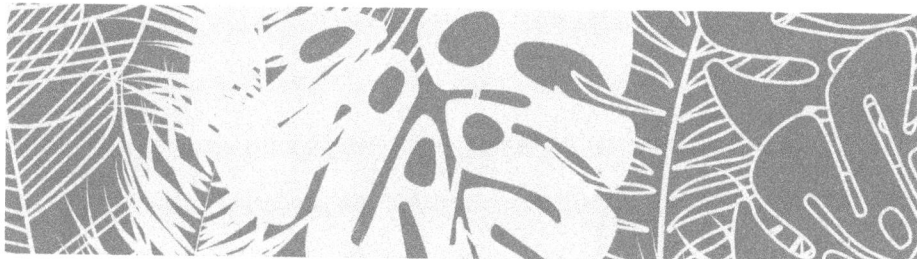

Low FODMAP
Food Diary

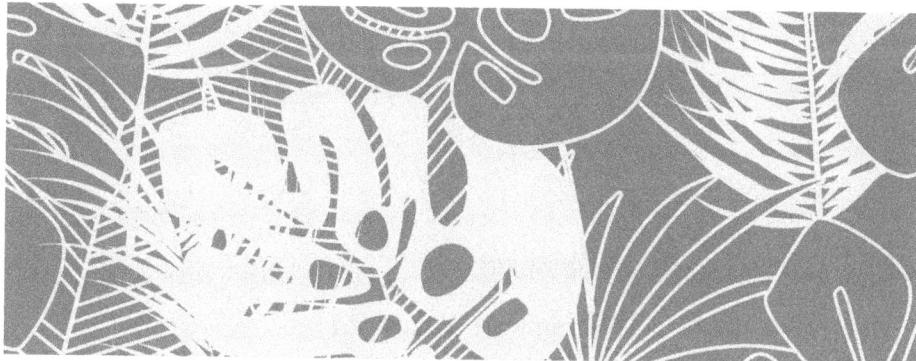

Daily Diary To Track Foods And Symptoms
To Beat IBS And Digestive Disorders

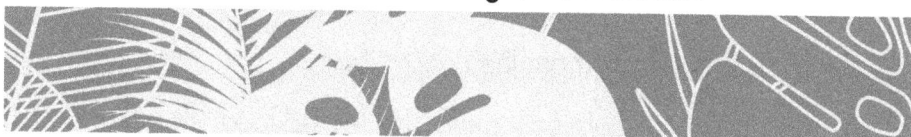

First published in 2018 by Erin Rose Publishing

Text and illustration copyright © 2018 Erin Rose Publishing

Design: Julie Anson

ISBN: 978-1-911492-77-1

A CIP record for this book is available from the British Library.

DISCLAIMER: This book is not intended as a substitute for the medical advice, diagnosis or treatment by a physician or qualified healthcare provider.

Introduction

Finding out which foods are causing your Irritable Bowel Syndrome can be confusing and the offending foods can be very different from person to person. To help you identify your trigger foods, we bring you this specially tailored IBS Food Diary. By using this book as your daily journal you can keep a complete essential record of all aspects of your diet together with symptomatic reactions making it easy for you to create your personal food diary. In this book there are sections for all the important information, so you can complete the sections quickly and easily, making gathering and organising your information simple!

Keeping this daily diary will give you a unique picture of your health, to improve your understanding of any negative reactions, so you can avoid IBS and digestive problems in the future. Your IBS diary helps you work towards discovering and completing 'Your Go-Ahead List'.

This IBS diet diary contains 3 months of journal pages for you to fill out and record your food intake and reactions on a daily basis, giving you a clear record of your digestive issues, helping you progress towards better health.

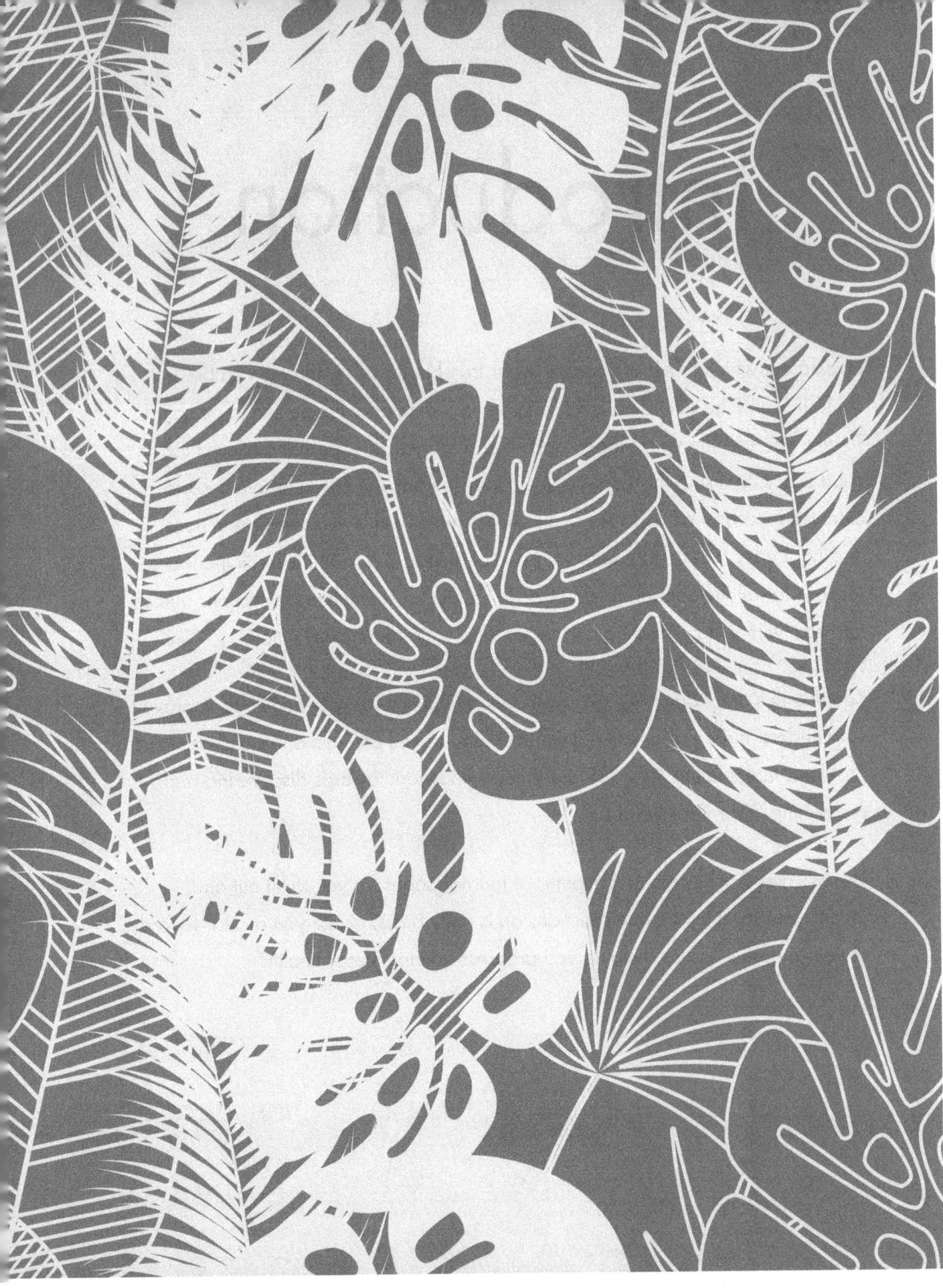

How To Use Your IBS Food Diary

This diary is easy to carry with you during the day so keep it handy if you are on-the-go.

Every time you eat or drink, write down in your daily food diary what you have consumed and then complete the comprehensive sections on Reaction, Fluid Intake, Mood and Bowel Action. Based on how your IBS or digestive disorder did or didn't react you can complete the section 'Symptom Description'.

By keeping your daily log you will be able to complete the section at the rear of this book to compile your own personal 'avoid' and 'go-ahead' list providing you with a valuable record of your unique dietary requirements.

Remember, if you have been avoiding a foodstuff for a period of time and re-introduce it at a later date you may be able to tolerate a small amount of that food. In this case you may be able to remove it from your 'Avoid' list and add it to your 'Go-Ahead' list or if you are in a re-introduction phase it may be helpful to complete a new diary which is up to date and can give you a helpful overview of your progress since you last sampled a food.

Wishing you great health!

Daily Food Diary

Date: . . . .

Time	🥣 Food & Quantity Consumed	Reaction: No ⊗ /Yes ✓

Symptoms Description	Scale 1-10

Stress Level (Tick one)		Fluid Intake	Bowel Action
😊			
😐			
☹️			

Daily Food Diary

Date: . . . .

Time	🍲 Food & Quantity Consumed	Reaction: No ✗/Yes ✓

Symptoms Description	Scale 1-10

Stress Level (Tick one)		Fluid Intake	Bowel Action
🙂			
😐			
☹️			

Daily Food Diary

Date: . . . .

Time	🍲 Food & Quantity Consumed	Reaction: No ⊗/Yes ✓

Symptoms Description	Scale 1-10

Stress Level (Tick one)		Fluid Intake	Bowel Action
☺			
😐			
☹			

Daily Food Diary

Date: . . . .

Time	🍲 Food & Quantity Consumed	Reaction: No ⊗/Yes ✓

Symptoms Description	Scale 1-10

Stress Level (Tick one)		Fluid Intake	Bowel Action
🙂			
😐			
☹️			

Daily Food Diary

Date: . . . .

Time	🍲 Food & Quantity Consumed	Reaction: No ✗ /Yes ✓

Symptoms Description	Scale 1-10

Stress Level (Tick one)		Fluid Intake	Bowel Action
🙂			
😐			
🙁			

Daily Food Diary

Date: . . . .

Time	🍲 Food & Quantity Consumed	Reaction: No ⊗/Yes ✓

Symptoms Description	Scale 1-10

Stress Level (Tick one)		Fluid Intake	Bowel Action
🙂			
😐			
☹️			

Daily Food Diary

Date: . . . .

Time	🍲 Food & Quantity Consumed	Reaction: No ✗/Yes ✓

Symptoms Description	Scale 1-10

Stress Level (Tick one)		Fluid Intake	Bowel Action
☺			
☹			
☹			

Daily Food Diary

Date: . . . .

Time	🍲 Food & Quantity Consumed	Reaction: No ⊗/Yes ✓

Symptoms Description	Scale 1-10

Stress Level (Tick one)		Fluid Intake	Bowel Action
☺			
😐			
☹			

Daily Food Diary

Date: ....

Time	🥣 Food & Quantity Consumed	Reaction: No ⊗ / Yes ✓

Symptoms Description	Scale 1-10

Stress Level (Tick one)		Fluid Intake	Bowel Action
☺			
😐			
☹			

Daily Food Diary

Date: . . . .

Time	🍲 Food & Quantity Consumed	Reaction: No ✗/Yes ✓

Symptoms Description	Scale 1-10

Stress Level (Tick one)	Fluid Intake	Bowel Action
☺		
😐		
☹		

Daily Food Diary

Date: . . . .

Time	🍲 Food & Quantity Consumed	Reaction: No ⊗ /Yes ✓

Symptoms Description	Scale 1-10

Stress Level (Tick one)		Fluid Intake	Bowel Action
🙂			
😐			
🙁			

Daily Food Diary

Date: . . . .

Time	🍲 Food & Quantity Consumed	Reaction: No ⊗/Yes ✓

Symptoms Description	Scale 1-10

Stress Level (Tick one)		Fluid Intake	Bowel Action
☺			
😐			
☹			

Daily Food Diary

Date: . . . .

Time	🍲 Food & Quantity Consumed	Reaction: No ✗ /Yes ✓

Symptoms Description	Scale 1-10

Stress Level (Tick one)		Fluid Intake	Bowel Action
☺			
😐			
☹			

Daily Food Diary

Date: . . . .

Time	🍲 Food & Quantity Consumed	Reaction: No ⊗ /Yes ✓

Symptoms Description	Scale 1-10

Stress Level (Tick one)		Fluid Intake	Bowel Action
☺			
😐			
☹			

Daily Food Diary

Date: . . . .

Time	🍲 Food & Quantity Consumed	Reaction: No ⊗/Yes ✓

Symptoms Description	Scale 1-10

Stress Level (Tick one)		Fluid Intake	Bowel Action
🙂			
😐			
🙁			

Daily Food Diary

Date: . . . .

Time	🍲 Food & Quantity Consumed	Reaction: No ⊗ / Yes ✓

Symptoms Description	Scale 1-10

Stress Level (Tick one)		Fluid Intake	Bowel Action
🙂			
😐			
☹️			

Daily Food Diary

Date: . . . .

Time	🍲 Food & Quantity Consumed	Reaction: No ⊗/Yes ✓

Symptoms Description	Scale 1-10

Stress Level (Tick one)		Fluid Intake	Bowel Action
🙂			
😐			
🙁			

Daily Food Diary

Date: . . . .

Time	🍲 Food & Quantity Consumed	Reaction: No ⊗/Yes ✓

Symptoms Description	Scale 1-10

Stress Level (Tick one)		Fluid Intake	Bowel Action
🙂			
😐			
☹️			

Daily Food Diary

Date: . . . .

Time	🍲 Food & Quantity Consumed	Reaction: No ⊗/Yes ✓

Symptoms Description	Scale 1-10

Stress Level (Tick one)		Fluid Intake	Bowel Action
🙂			
😐			
🙁			

Daily Food Diary

Date: . . . .

Time	🍲 Food & Quantity Consumed	Reaction: No ⊗ / Yes ✓

Symptoms Description	Scale 1-10

Stress Level (Tick one)		Fluid Intake	Bowel Action
☺			
☹			
☹			

Daily Food Diary

Date: . . . .

Time	🥣 Food & Quantity Consumed	Reaction: No ✗/Yes ✓

Symptoms Description	Scale 1-10

Stress Level (Tick one)		Fluid Intake	Bowel Action
☺			
☹			
☹			

Daily Food Diary

Date: . . . .

Time	🍲 Food & Quantity Consumed	Reaction: No⊗/Yes✓

Symptoms Description	Scale 1-10

Stress Level (Tick one)		Fluid Intake	Bowel Action
☺			
😐			
☹			

Daily Food Diary

Date: . . . .

Time	🍲 Food & Quantity Consumed	Reaction: No ✗/Yes ✓

Symptoms Description	Scale 1-10

Stress Level (Tick one)		Fluid Intake	Bowel Action
🙂			
😐			
🙁			

Daily Food Diary

Date: . . . .

Time	🍲 Food & Quantity Consumed	Reaction: No ⊗ /Yes ✓

Symptoms Description	Scale 1-10

Stress Level (Tick one)		Fluid Intake	Bowel Action
☺			
😐			
☹			

Daily Food Diary

Date: . . . .

Time	🍲 Food & Quantity Consumed	Reaction: No ⊗/Yes ✓

Symptoms Description	Scale 1-10

Stress Level (Tick one)		Fluid Intake	Bowel Action
☺			
☹			
☹			

Daily Food Diary

Date: . . . .

Time	🍜 Food & Quantity Consumed	Reaction: No ⊗/Yes ✓

Symptoms Description	Scale 1-10

Stress Level (Tick one)		Fluid Intake	Bowel Action
😊			
😐			
☹️			

Daily Food Diary

Date: . . . .

Time	🍲 Food & Quantity Consumed	Reaction: No ✖ /Yes ✔

Symptoms Description	Scale 1-10

Stress Level (Tick one)		Fluid Intake	Bowel Action
🙂			
😐			
🙁			

Daily Food Diary

Date: . . . .

Time	🍲 Food & Quantity Consumed	Reaction: No ⊗/Yes ✓

Symptoms Description	Scale 1-10

Stress Level (Tick one)		Fluid Intake	Bowel Action
🙂			
😐			
🙁			

Daily Food Diary

Date: . . . .

Time	🍲 Food & Quantity Consumed	Reaction: No ✗/Yes ✓

Symptoms Description	Scale 1-10

Stress Level (Tick one)		Fluid Intake	Bowel Action
☺			
☹			
☹			

Daily Food Diary

Date: . . . .

Time	🍲 Food & Quantity Consumed	Reaction: No ✗/Yes ✓

Symptoms Description	Scale 1-10

Stress Level (Tick one)		Fluid Intake	Bowel Action
🙂			
😐			
🙁			

Daily Food Diary

Date: . . . .

Time	🍲 Food & Quantity Consumed	Reaction: No ⊗ /Yes ✓

Symptoms Description	Scale 1-10

Stress Level (Tick one)		Fluid Intake	Bowel Action
😊			
😐			
☹			

Daily Food Diary

Date: . . . .

Time	🍲 Food & Quantity Consumed	Reaction: No ⊗/Yes ✓

Symptoms Description	Scale 1-10

Stress Level (Tick one)		Fluid Intake	Bowel Action
☺			
😐			
☹			

Daily Food Diary

Date: . . . .

Time	🍲 Food & Quantity Consumed	Reaction: No ⊗/Yes ✓

Symptoms Description	Scale 1-10

Stress Level (Tick one)		Fluid Intake	Bowel Action
☺			
☹			
☹			

Daily Food Diary

Date: . . . .

Time	🍲 Food & Quantity Consumed	Reaction: No ⊗/Yes ✓

Symptoms Description	Scale 1-10

Stress Level (Tick one)		Fluid Intake	Bowel Action
🙂			
😐			
☹️			

Daily Food Diary

Date: . . . .

Time	🍲 Food & Quantity Consumed	Reaction: No❌/Yes✅

Symptoms Description	Scale 1-10

Stress Level (Tick one)	Fluid Intake	Bowel Action
🙂		
😐		
☹️		

Daily Food Diary

Date: . . . .

Time	🍲 Food & Quantity Consumed	Reaction: No ✗ / Yes ✓

Symptoms Description	Scale 1-10

Stress Level (Tick one)		Fluid Intake	Bowel Action
☺			
😐			
☹			

Daily Food Diary

Date: . . . .

Time	🍲 Food & Quantity Consumed	Reaction: No ⊗/Yes ✓

Symptoms Description	Scale 1-10

Stress Level (Tick one)		Fluid Intake	Bowel Action
🙂			
😐			
☹️			

Daily Food Diary

Date: . . . .

Time	🍲 Food & Quantity Consumed	Reaction: No ⊗/Yes ✓

Symptoms Description	Scale 1-10

Stress Level (Tick one)		Fluid Intake	Bowel Action
☺			
😐			
☹			

Daily Food Diary

Date: . . . .

Time	🍲 Food & Quantity Consumed	Reaction: No ✗/Yes ✓

Symptoms Description	Scale 1-10

Stress Level (Tick one)		Fluid Intake	Bowel Action
☺			
😐			
☹			

Daily Food Diary

Date: . . . .

Time	🍲 Food & Quantity Consumed	Reaction: No⊗/Yes✓

Symptoms Description	Scale 1-10

Stress Level (Tick one)		Fluid Intake	Bowel Action
🙂			
😐			
🙁			

Daily Food Diary

Date: ....

Time	🍲 Food & Quantity Consumed	Reaction: No ⊗ / Yes ✓

Symptoms Description	Scale 1-10

Stress Level (Tick one)		Fluid Intake	Bowel Action
🙂			
😐			
☹️			

Daily Food Diary

Date: . . . .

Time	🥣 Food & Quantity Consumed	Reaction: No ⊗/Yes ✓

Symptoms Description	Scale 1-10

Stress Level (Tick one)		Fluid Intake	Bowel Action
🙂			
😐			
🙁			

Daily Food Diary

Date: . . . .

Time	🍲 Food & Quantity Consumed	Reaction: No ❌/Yes ✅

Symptoms Description	Scale 1-10

Stress Level (Tick one)		Fluid Intake	Bowel Action
☺			
😐			
☹			

Daily Food Diary

Date: . . . .

Time	🍲 Food & Quantity Consumed	Reaction: No ⊗/Yes ✓

Symptoms Description	Scale 1-10

Stress Level (Tick one)		Fluid Intake	Bowel Action
☺			
😐			
☹			

Daily Food Diary

Date: . . . .

Time	🍲 Food & Quantity Consumed	Reaction: No ⊗/Yes ✓

Symptoms Description	Scale 1-10

Stress Level (Tick one)		Fluid Intake	Bowel Action
☺			
☹			
☹			

Daily Food Diary

Date: . . . .

Time	🍲 Food & Quantity Consumed	Reaction: No ⊗ /Yes ✓

Symptoms Description	Scale 1-10

Stress Level (Tick one)		Fluid Intake	Bowel Action
😊			
😐			
☹			

Daily Food Diary

Date: . . . .

Time	🍲 Food & Quantity Consumed	Reaction: No ✗ /Yes ✓

Symptoms Description	Scale 1-10

Stress Level (Tick one)		Fluid Intake	Bowel Action
🙂			
😐			
☹️			

Daily Food Diary

Date: . . . .

Time	🍲 Food & Quantity Consumed	Reaction: No ✗/Yes ✓

Symptoms Description	Scale 1-10

Stress Level (Tick one)		Fluid Intake	Bowel Action
☺			
😐			
☹			

Daily Food Diary

Date: . . . .

Time	🥣 Food & Quantity Consumed	Reaction: No ⊗/Yes ✓

Symptoms Description	Scale 1-10

Stress Level (Tick one)		Fluid Intake	Bowel Action
🙂			
😐			
☹️			

Daily Food Diary

Date: . . . .

Time	🍲 Food & Quantity Consumed	Reaction: No ✗/Yes ✓

Symptoms Description	Scale 1-10

Stress Level (Tick one)		Fluid Intake	Bowel Action
🙂			
😐			
🙁			

Daily Food Diary

Date: . . . .

Time	🍲 Food & Quantity Consumed	Reaction: No ⊗ /Yes ✓

Symptoms Description	Scale 1-10

Stress Level (Tick one)	Fluid Intake	Bowel Action
☺		
😐		
☹		

Daily Food Diary

Date: . . . .

Time	🍲 Food & Quantity Consumed	Reaction: No ✗/Yes ✓

Symptoms Description	Scale 1-10

Stress Level (Tick one)		Fluid Intake	Bowel Action
🙂			
😐			
🙁			

Daily Food Diary

Date: . . . .

Time	🍲 Food & Quantity Consumed	Reaction: No ⊗ / Yes ✓

Symptoms Description	Scale 1-10

Stress Level (Tick one)		Fluid Intake	Bowel Action
☺			
☹			
☹			

Daily Food Diary

Date: . . . .

Time	🍲 Food & Quantity Consumed	Reaction: No ⊗/Yes ✓

Symptoms Description	Scale 1-10

Stress Level (Tick one)		Fluid Intake	Bowel Action
☺			
😐			
☹			

Daily Food Diary

Date: . . . .

Time	🥣 Food & Quantity Consumed	Reaction: No ✗ /Yes ✓

Symptoms Description	Scale 1-10

Stress Level (Tick one)		Fluid Intake	Bowel Action
☺			
😐			
☹			

Daily Food Diary

Date: . . . .

Time	🍲 Food & Quantity Consumed	Reaction: No ⊗/Yes ✓

Symptoms Description	Scale 1-10

Stress Level (Tick one)		Fluid Intake	Bowel Action
☺			
😐			
☹			

Daily Food Diary

Date: . . . .

Time	🍲 Food & Quantity Consumed	Reaction: No ⊗/Yes ✓

Symptoms Description	Scale 1-10

Stress Level (Tick one)		Fluid Intake	Bowel Action
☺			
😐			
☹			

Daily Food Diary

Date: . . . .

Time	🥣 Food & Quantity Consumed	Reaction: No ⊗ /Yes ✓

Symptoms Description	Scale 1-10

Stress Level (Tick one)		Fluid Intake	Bowel Action
🙂			
😐			
☹️			

Daily Food Diary

Date: . . . .

Time	🍲 Food & Quantity Consumed	Reaction: No ⊗ /Yes ✓

Symptoms Description	Scale 1-10

Stress Level (Tick one)		Fluid Intake	Bowel Action
☺			
😐			
☹			

Daily Food Diary

Date: . . . .

Time	🍲 Food & Quantity Consumed	Reaction: No ⊗/Yes ✓

Symptoms Description	Scale 1-10

Stress Level (Tick one)		Fluid Intake	Bowel Action
☺			
😐			
☹			

Daily Food Diary

Date: . . . .

Time	🍲 Food & Quantity Consumed	Reaction: No ⊗ /Yes ✓

Symptoms Description	Scale 1-10

Stress Level (Tick one)		Fluid Intake	Bowel Action
☺			
☹			
☹			

Daily Food Diary

Date: . . . .

Time	🥣 Food & Quantity Consumed	Reaction: No ⊗/Yes ✓

Symptoms Description	Scale 1-10

Stress Level (Tick one)		Fluid Intake	Bowel Action
🙂			
😐			
☹️			

Daily Food Diary

Date: . . . .

Time	🍲 Food & Quantity Consumed	Reaction: No ⊗ /Yes ✓

Symptoms Description	Scale 1-10

Stress Level (Tick one)		Fluid Intake	Bowel Action
🙂			
😐			
🙁			

Daily Food Diary

Date: . . . .

Time	🍜 Food & Quantity Consumed	Reaction: No ⊗/Yes ✓

Symptoms Description	Scale 1-10

Stress Level (Tick one)		Fluid Intake	Bowel Action
🙂			
😐			
🙁			

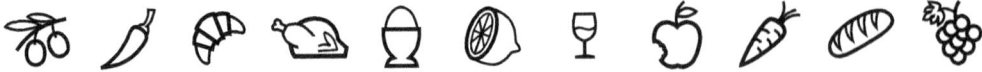

Daily Food Diary

Date: . . . .

Time	🥣 Food & Quantity Consumed	Reaction: No ⊗/Yes ✓

Symptoms Description	Scale 1-10

Stress Level (Tick one)		Fluid Intake	Bowel Action
☺			
☹			
☹			

Daily Food Diary

Date: . . . .

Time	🍲 Food & Quantity Consumed	Reaction: No ⊗ /Yes ✓

Symptoms Description	Scale 1-10

Stress Level (Tick one)		Fluid Intake	Bowel Action
☺			
😐			
☹			

Daily Food Diary

Date: . . . .

Time	🍲 Food & Quantity Consumed	Reaction: No ✗/Yes ✓

Symptoms Description	Scale 1-10

Stress Level (Tick one)		Fluid Intake	Bowel Action
☺			
😐			
☹			

Daily Food Diary

Date: . . . .

Time	🥣 Food & Quantity Consumed	Reaction: No ⊗ / Yes ✓

Symptoms Description	Scale 1-10

Stress Level (Tick one)		Fluid Intake	Bowel Action
☺			
☹			
☹			

Daily Food Diary

Date: . . . .

Time	🍲 Food & Quantity Consumed	Reaction: No ⊗ /Yes ✓

Symptoms Description	Scale 1-10

Stress Level (Tick one)		Fluid Intake	Bowel Action
🙂			
😐			
🙁			

Daily Food Diary

Date: . . . .

Time	🍲 Food & Quantity Consumed	Reaction: No ⊗/Yes ✓

Symptoms Description	Scale 1-10

Stress Level (Tick one)		Fluid Intake	Bowel Action
🙂			
😐			
🙁			

Daily Food Diary

Date: . . . .

Time	🍲 Food & Quantity Consumed	Reaction: No ✗/Yes ✓

Symptoms Description	Scale 1-10

Stress Level (Tick one)		Fluid Intake	Bowel Action
🙂			
😐			
🙁			

Daily Food Diary

Date: . . . .

Time	🍲 Food & Quantity Consumed	Reaction: No ⊗/Yes ✓

Symptoms Description	Scale 1-10

Stress Level (Tick one)		Fluid Intake	Bowel Action
🙂			
😐			
🙁			

Daily Food Diary

Date: ....

Time	🍲 Food & Quantity Consumed	Reaction: No ⊗/Yes ✓

Symptoms Description	Scale 1-10

Stress Level (Tick one)		Fluid Intake	Bowel Action
😊			
😐			
☹️			

Daily Food Diary

Date: . . . .

Time	🍲 Food & Quantity Consumed	Reaction: No ⊗ /Yes ✓

Symptoms Description	Scale 1-10

Stress Level (Tick one)		Fluid Intake	Bowel Action
😊			
😐			
☹️			

Daily Food Diary

Date: . . . .

Time	🍲 Food & Quantity Consumed	Reaction: No ⊗ / Yes ✓

Symptoms Description	Scale 1-10

Stress Level (Tick one)		Fluid Intake	Bowel Action
🙂			
😐			
☹️			

Daily Food Diary

Date: . . . .

Time	🍲 Food & Quantity Consumed	Reaction: No ✕/Yes ✓

Symptoms Description	Scale 1-10

Stress Level (Tick one)		Fluid Intake	Bowel Action
☺			
😐			
☹			

Daily Food Diary

Date: . . . .

Time	🍲 Food & Quantity Consumed	Reaction: No ⊗/Yes ✓

Symptoms Description	Scale 1-10

Stress Level (Tick one)		Fluid Intake	Bowel Action
☺			
😐			
☹			

Daily Food Diary

Date: . . . .

Time	🍲 Food & Quantity Consumed	Reaction: No ⊗ / Yes ✓

Symptoms Description	Scale 1-10

Stress Level (Tick one)		Fluid Intake	Bowel Action
🙂			
😐			
☹️			

Daily Food Diary

Date: . . . .

Time	🍲 Food & Quantity Consumed	Reaction: No ⊗/Yes ✓

Symptoms Description	Scale 1-10

Stress Level (Tick one)		Fluid Intake	Bowel Action
☺			
😐			
☹			

Daily Food Diary

Date: . . . .

Time	🥣 Food & Quantity Consumed	Reaction: No ⊗ / Yes ✓

Symptoms Description	Scale 1-10

Stress Level (Tick one)		Fluid Intake	Bowel Action
☺			
☹			
☹			

Daily Food Diary

Date: ....

Time	🍲 Food & Quantity Consumed	Reaction: No ⊗/Yes ✓

Symptoms Description	Scale 1-10

Stress Level (Tick one)		Fluid Intake	Bowel Action
☺			
☹			
☹			

Daily Food Diary

Date: . . . .

Time	🥣 Food & Quantity Consumed	Reaction: No ⊗ /Yes ✓

Symptoms Description	Scale 1-10

Stress Level (Tick one)		Fluid Intake	Bowel Action
🙂			
😐			
☹️			

Daily Food Diary

Date: . . . .

Time	🍚 Food & Quantity Consumed	Reaction: No⊗/Yes✓

Symptoms Description	Scale 1-10

Stress Level (Tick one)		Fluid Intake	Bowel Action
🙂			
😐			
☹️			

Daily Food Diary

Date: . . . .

Time	🍲 Food & Quantity Consumed	Reaction: No ⊗/Yes ✓

Symptoms Description	Scale 1-10

Stress Level (Tick one)		Fluid Intake	Bowel Action
☺			
😐			
☹			

Daily Food Diary

Date: . . . .

Time	🍲 Food & Quantity Consumed	Reaction: No ✗ / Yes ✓

Symptoms Description	Scale 1-10

Stress Level (Tick one)		Fluid Intake	Bowel Action
☺			
😐			
☹			

Daily Food Diary

Date: . . . .

Time	🥣 Food & Quantity Consumed	Reaction: No ⊗/Yes ✓

Symptoms Description	Scale 1-10

Stress Level (Tick one)		Fluid Intake	Bowel Action
😊			
😐			
☹			

Daily Food Diary

Date: . . . .

Time	🍲 Food & Quantity Consumed	Reaction: No ⊗ /Yes ✓

Symptoms Description	Scale 1-10

Stress Level (Tick one)		Fluid Intake	Bowel Action
😊			
😐			
☹			

Daily Food Diary

Date: . . . .

Time	🍲 Food & Quantity Consumed	Reaction: No ⊗/Yes ✓

Symptoms Description	Scale 1-10

Stress Level (Tick one)	Fluid Intake	Bowel Action
☺		
😐		
☹		

Daily Food Diary

Date: . . . .

Time	🍲 Food & Quantity Consumed	Reaction: No ✗ / Yes ✓

Symptoms Description	Scale 1-10

Stress Level (Tick one)		Fluid Intake	Bowel Action
🙂			
😐			
☹️			

Daily Food Diary

Date: . . . .

Time	🍲 Food & Quantity Consumed	Reaction: No ⊗/Yes ✓

Symptoms Description	Scale 1-10

Stress Level (Tick one)		Fluid Intake	Bowel Action
🙂			
😐			
☹️			

(X) Your Personal AVOID list

Quantity	Food	Symptoms caused Scale 1-10	Date

(X) Your Personal AVOID list

Quantity	Food	Symptoms caused Scale 1-10	Date

✖ Your Personal AVOID list

Quantity	Food	Symptoms caused Scale 1-10	Date

✓ Your Personal GO AHEAD list

Quantity	Food	Date

✔ Your Personal GO AHEAD list

Quantity	Food	Date

✓ Your Personal GO AHEAD list

Quantity	Food	Date

You may also be interested in other titles by
Erin Rose Publishing
which are available in both paperback and ebook.

⏱ **Quick Start Guides**

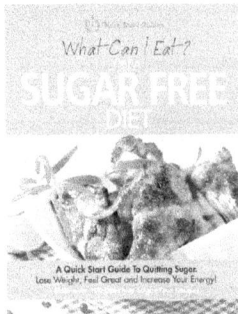

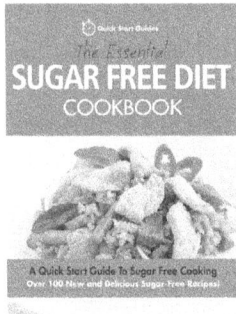

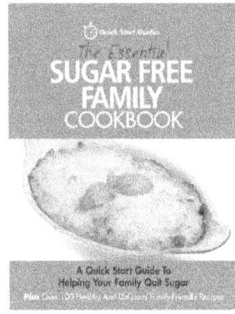

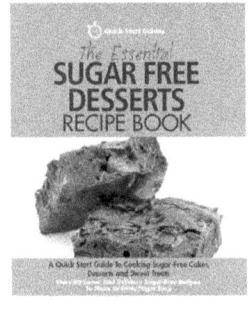

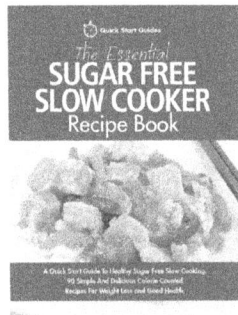

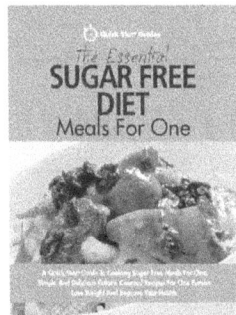

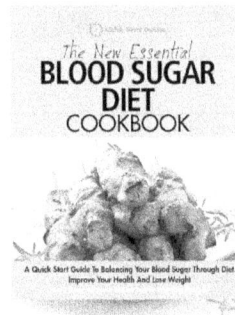

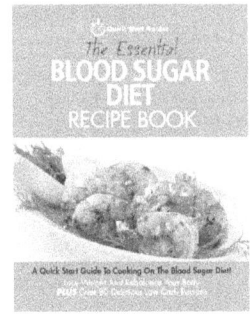

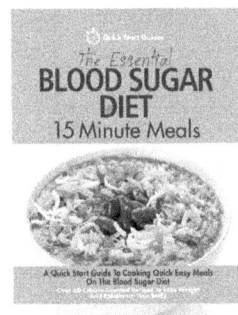

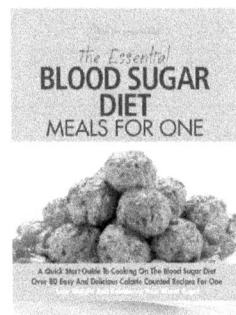

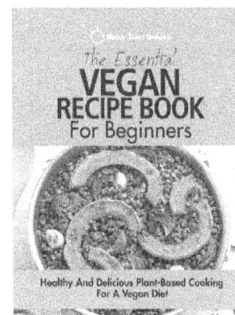

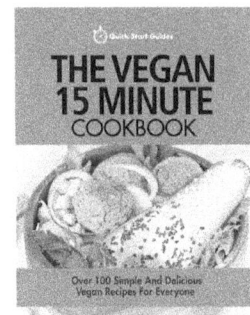

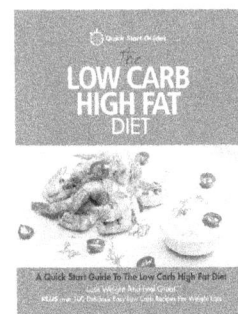

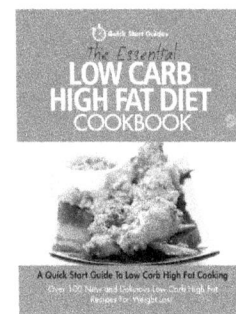

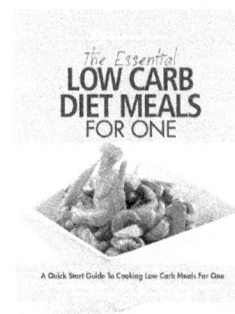

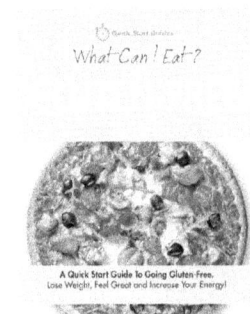

What Can I Eat? **SUGAR FREE** DIET A Quick Start Guide To Quitting Sugar. Lose Weight, Feel Great and Increase Your Energy!	**SUGAR FREE DIET** COOKBOOK A Quick Start Guide To Sugar Free Cooking Over 100 New and Delicious Sugar Free Recipes!	The Essential **SUGAR FREE FAMILY** COOKBOOK A Quick Start Guide To Helping Your Family Quit Sugar	The Essential **SUGAR FREE DESSERTS** RECIPE BOOK A Quick Start Guide To Cooking Sugar Free Cakes, Desserts and Sweet Treats
SUGAR FREE SLOW COOKER Recipe Book A Quick Start Guide To Healthy Sugar Free Slow Cooking. 90 Simple And Delicious Calorie Counted Recipes For Weight Loss and Good Health	The Essential **SUGAR FREE DIET** Meals For One	The New Essential **BLOOD SUGAR DIET** COOKBOOK A Quick Start Guide To Balancing Your Blood Sugar Through Diet. Improve Your Health And Lose Weight	The Essential **BLOOD SUGAR DIET** RECIPE BOOK A Quick Start Guide To Cooking On The Blood Sugar Diet
The Essential **BLOOD SUGAR DIET** 15 Minute Meals	The Essential **BLOOD SUGAR DIET** MEALS FOR ONE	The Essential **VEGAN RECIPE BOOK** For Beginners Healthy And Delicious Plant-Based Cooking For A Vegan Diet!	**THE VEGAN 15 MINUTE** COOKBOOK Over 100 Simple And Delicious Vegan Recipes For Everyone
LOW CARB HIGH FAT DIET A Quick Start Guide To The Low Carb High Fat Diet	The Essential **LOW CARB HIGH FAT DIET** COOKBOOK A Quick Start Guide To Low Carb High Fat Cooking Over 100 New and Delicious Low Carb High Fat Recipes For Weight Loss!	The Essential **LOW CARB DIET MEALS** FOR ONE A Quick Start Guide To Cooking Low Carb Meals For One	What Can I Eat? A Quick Start Guide To Going Gluten-free. Lose Weight, Feel Great and Increase Your Energy!

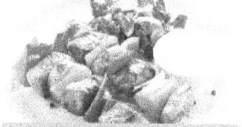

The Essential
HEALTHY GUT DIET RECIPE BOOK

A Quick Start Guide To Improving Your Digestion, Health And Wellbeing

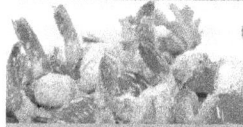

The Essential
Low FODMAP Diet COOKBOOK

A Quick Start Guide To Relieving the Symptoms of IBS Through Diet

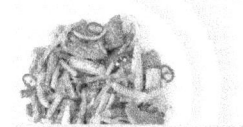

The Essential
DIABETES DIET COOKBOOK

A Quick Start Guide To Managing Your Diabetes Through Diet

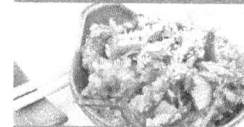

The
ALKALINE DIET SOLUTION

A Quick Start Guide To The Alkaline Diet

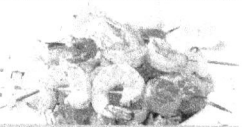

The Essential
THYROID DIET RECIPE BOOK

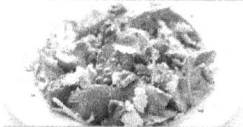

The Essential
SIRT FOOD DIET RECIPE BOOK

A Quick Start Guide to Cooking on the SIRT Food Diet!

What Can I Eat? ON A
DAIRY FREE DIET

A Quick Start Guide To Quitting Dairy and Lactose

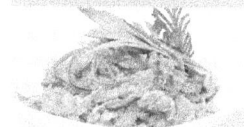

LOWER CHOLESTEROL DIET

A Quick Start Guide To Lower Cholesterol

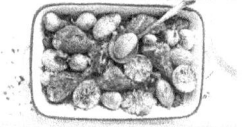

The Essential
ROASTING TIN COOKBOOK

Over 80 Easy And Delicious One Dish, No-Fuss Oven Recipes

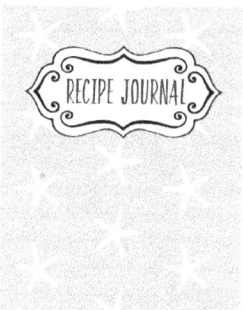

RECIPE JOURNAL

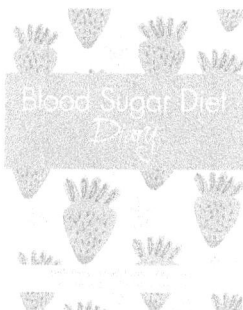

Blood Sugar Diet Diary

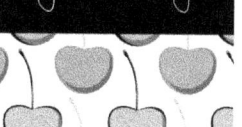

My Diet Diary

Daily Diet, Health, And Fitness Diary To Track Weight Loss and Well-being

Low FODMAP Diet Diary

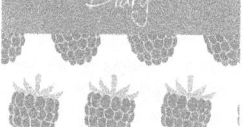

Sugar-Free Diet Diary

FOOD Diary

www.ingramcontent.com/pod-product-compliance
Lightning Source LLC
Chambersburg PA
CBHW081257040426
42452CB00014B/2539